D1639647

WITHDRAWN
SWANSEA LIBRARIES

6000303523

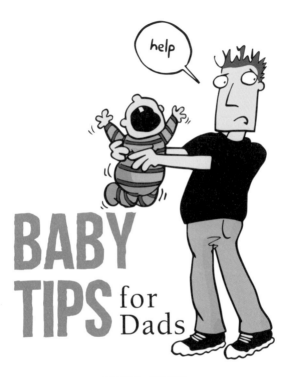

BABY
TIPS for
Dads

SIMON BRETT

Illustrations by Alex Hallatt

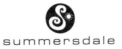

summersdale

BABY TIPS FOR DADS

First published in 2004
Reprinted 2005, 2006, 2007 and 2012

Illustrations by Alex Hallatt

Summersdale Publishers Ltd
46 West Street
Chichester
West Sussex
PO19 1RP
UK

www.summersdale.com

Printed and bound in China

ISBN: 978-1-78685-045-4

Substantial discounts on bulk quantities of Summersdale books are available to corporations, professional associations and other organisations. For details contact general enquiries: telephone: +44 (0) 1243 771107, fax: +44 (0) 1243 786300 or email: enquiries@summersdale.com.

TO...................................

FROM...............................

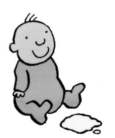

CONTENTS

INTRODUCTION

So there it is – your very own little baby. You are a dad. What a wonderful achievement! Granted, your partner may have made a greater contribution to the whole process, but your input was at least as important as hers – and a lot more fun.

So, how are you going to cope with this new presence in your household? No amount of antenatal classes or concentrated reading of childcare manuals can prepare you for the reality of a baby. This little book, however, will give you some useful tips on how to face the challenges ahead.

HOW TO PLAY THE PERFECT PARTNER

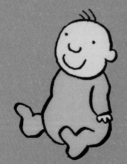

THINGS TO SAY TO YOUR PARTNER AFTER SHE'S HAD A BABY:

'You've done enough by having the baby – I'll do everything else.' (It's a very tactful wheeze to say this. Doing it is a different matter entirely.)

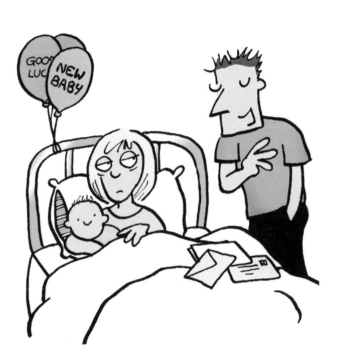

THINGS TO SAY TO YOUR PARTNER AFTER SHE'S HAD A BABY:

'I really think you look thinner since you've had the baby.'

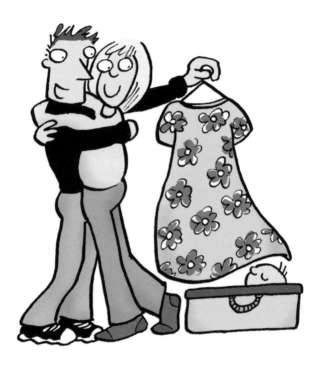

THINGS TO SAY TO YOUR PARTNER AFTER SHE'S HAD A BABY:

'I'll be happy to babysit whenever you want to go out for a girly night with your friends.'

THINGS TO SAY TO YOUR PARTNER AFTER SHE'S HAD A BABY:

'You need your sleep. I'll go into the spare room next to the nursery, and I'll get up if the baby wakes in the night.'

THINGS TO SAY TO YOUR PARTNER AFTER SHE'S HAD A BABY:

'Don't worry about me – we'll get our sex life back on track when you feel like it. No hurry.'

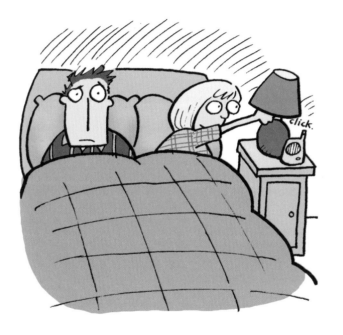

THINGS TO SAY TO YOUR PARTNER AFTER SHE'S HAD A BABY:

'We'll get an au pair.'

THINGS NOT TO SAY TO YOUR PARTNER AFTER SHE'S HAD A BABY:

'Ooh look – a stretch-mark!'

'Phwoar, look at that woman over there – her stomach's like an ironing board.'

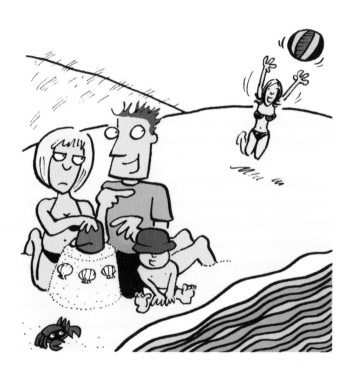

THINGS NOT TO SAY TO YOUR PARTNER AFTER SHE'S HAD A BABY:

'The baby's birth was relatively easy.'

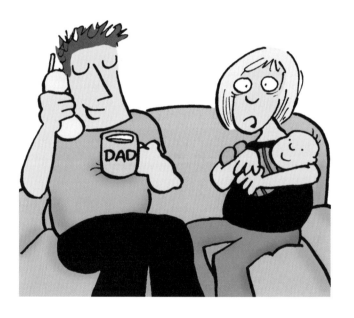

THINGS NOT TO SAY TO YOUR PARTNER AFTER SHE'S HAD A BABY:

'I don't think you've got very much fatter.'

THINGS NOT TO SAY TO YOUR PARTNER AFTER SHE'S HAD A BABY:

'You always did have good child-bearing hips.'

THINGS NOT TO SAY TO YOUR PARTNER AFTER SHE'S HAD A BABY:

'She's not with me.' (Said when your partner starts breastfeeding in public.)

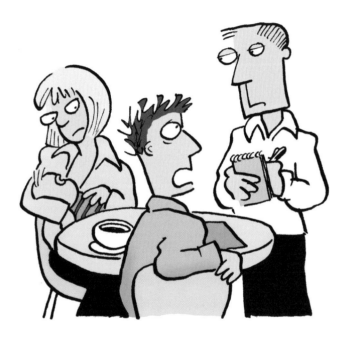

THINGS NOT TO SAY TO YOUR PARTNER AFTER SHE'S HAD A BABY:

'No one expects a woman's breasts to be quite so firm and pert after she's had a baby.'

AND DON'T SAY THIS ONE AT ANY TIME:

'You are getting to look more and more like your mother.'

SIGNS YOUR PARTNER IS SPENDING TOO MUCH TIME WITH THE BABY:

Every time she drives you anywhere there are nursery rhymes playing in the car – and you're expected to join in with them.

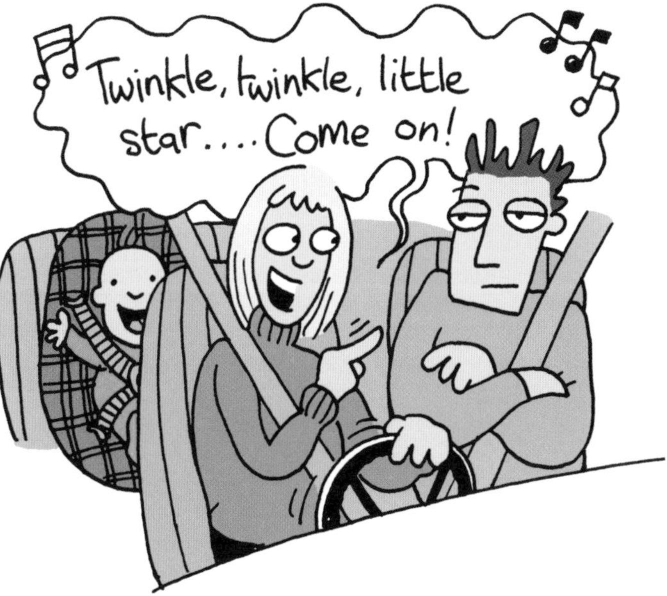
Twinkle, twinkle, little star.... Come on!

SIGNS YOUR PARTNER IS SPENDING TOO MUCH TIME WITH THE BABY:

Everybody gets a bib
at dinner time.

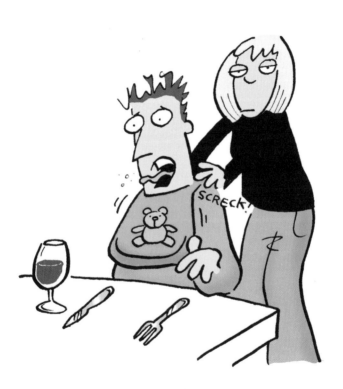

SIGNS YOUR PARTNER IS SPENDING TOO MUCH TIME WITH THE BABY:

She cuts up the food of the person next to her at a dinner party.

ALWAYS AGREE:

When your partner says
your baby is prettier/more
intelligent/more advanced
than anyone else's baby.

ALWAYS AGREE:

That your baby looks exactly like whichever relative happens to be in the room at any given moment.

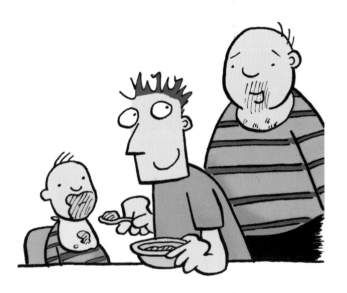

ALWAYS AGREE:

With your mother-in-law. Well, at least try! Unless of course you're in the room when your partner and mother-in-law are discussing childcare and want you to take sides. In that case, go down the pub.

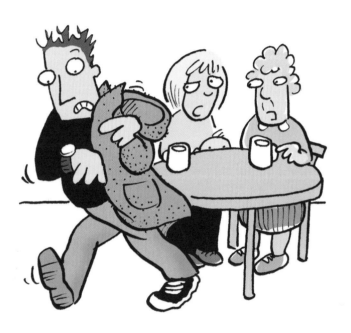

ALWAYS AGREE:

With your partner's views on childcare (so long as they don't involve you doing too much).

DADDY DOS AND DON'TS

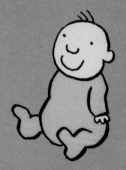

UNDER NO CIRCUMSTANCES BE HEARD TO SAY ANY OF THE FOLLOWING (YOU'LL REGRET IT IF YOU DO):

'The baby's going to have to fit into our routine.'

'I will never allow any baby of mine to...' (Fill in the blank. Whatever you say, of course you will.)

UNDER NO CIRCUMSTANCES
BE HEARD TO SAY ANY
OF THE FOLLOWING:

'The baby's never
been carsick.'

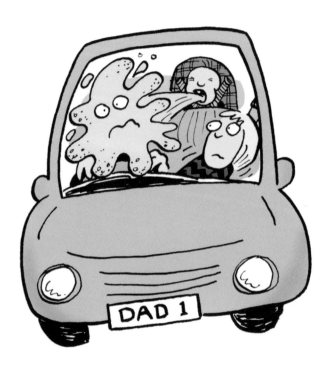

UNDER NO CIRCUMSTANCES BE HEARD TO SAY ANY OF THE FOLLOWING:

'We've been very lucky with the baby sleeping through the night.'

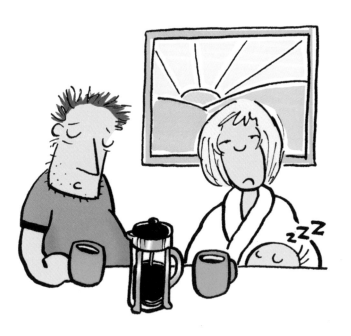

UNDER NO CIRCUMSTANCES BE HEARD TO SAY ANY OF THE FOLLOWING:

'We're certainly not going to let having a baby affect our sex life.'

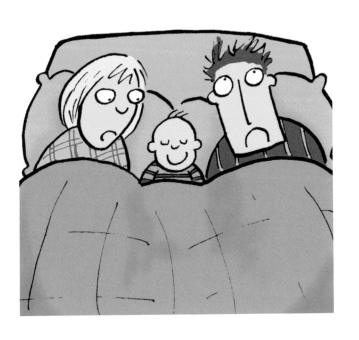

UNDER NO CIRCUMSTANCES BE HEARD TO SAY ANY OF THE FOLLOWING:

'I don't know why people make such a big deal about having a baby.'

TRY TO SEE THINGS FROM YOUR BABY'S POINT OF VIEW. THEN YOU WILL UNDERSTAND THAT:

The sole purpose of your eyes is to have fingers poked into them.

TRY TO SEE THINGS FROM YOUR
BABY'S POINT OF VIEW. THEN
YOU WILL UNDERSTAND THAT:

The sole purpose of your
hair is to have baby food
mashed into it.

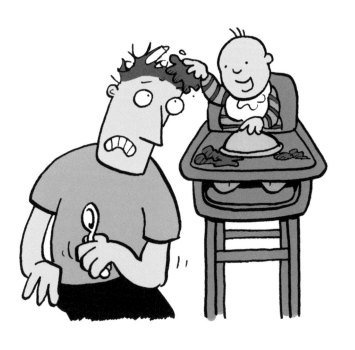

TRY TO SEE THINGS FROM YOUR BABY'S POINT OF VIEW. THEN YOU WILL UNDERSTAND THAT:

The sole purpose of your clothes is for them to be puked over.

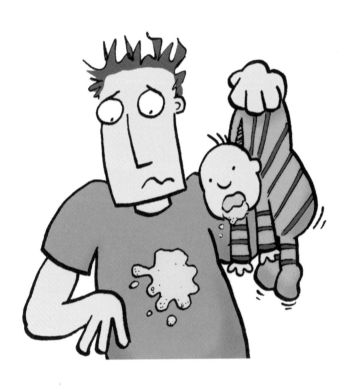

YOUR BABY REGARDS IT AS A SOLEMN DUTY TO STOP YOU FROM DOING ANY OF THE FOLLOWING:

Forgetting for a moment that you have a baby.

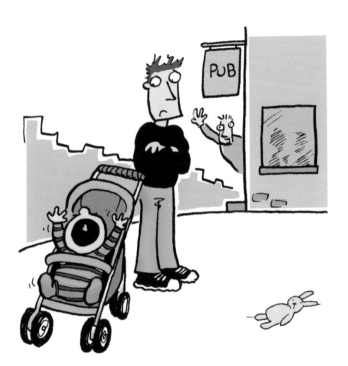

YOUR BABY REGARDS IT AS A SOLEMN DUTY TO STOP YOU FROM DOING ANY OF THE FOLLOWING:

Getting its clothes on.

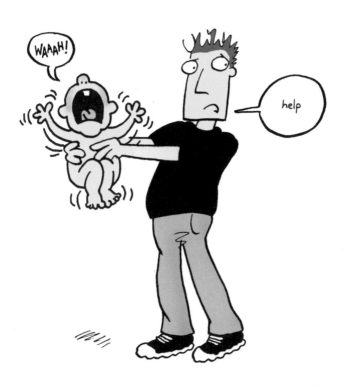

YOUR BABY REGARDS IT AS A SOLEMN DUTY TO STOP YOU FROM DOING ANY OF THE FOLLOWING:

Getting its nappy on.

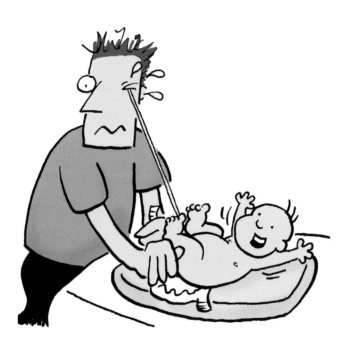

YOUR BABY REGARDS IT AS A SOLEMN DUTY TO STOP YOU FROM DOING ANY OF THE FOLLOWING:

Having a social life.

YOUR BABY REGARDS IT AS A SOLEMN DUTY TO STOP YOU FROM DOING ANY OF THE FOLLOWING:

Having a sex life.

YOUR BABY REGARDS IT AS A SOLEMN DUTY TO STOP YOU FROM DOING ANY OF THE FOLLOWING:

Sleeping.

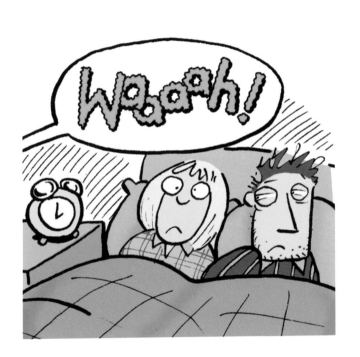

BABY PROVERBS FOR NEW DADS

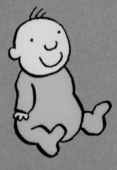

BABY PROVERBS FOR NEW DADS:

What you lose on the swings you lose on the roundabouts – you have to keep on pushing on both of them.

BABY PROVERBS FOR NEW DADS:

Cleanliness is next
to impossible.

BABY PROVERBS FOR NEW DADS:

People who live in glass houses with babies have very smeary windows.

BABY PROVERBS FOR NEW DADS:

A bad father blames
his tool.

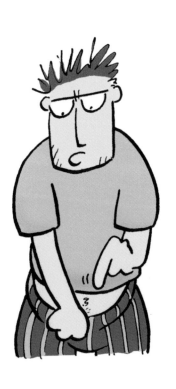

BABY PROVERBS FOR NEW DADS:

The early baby catches the worm... and then eats it.

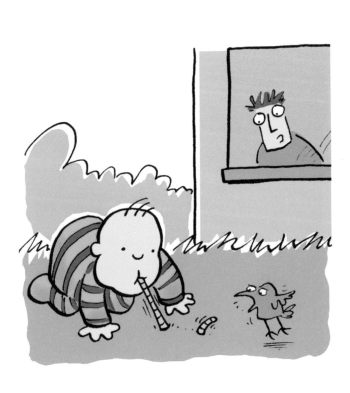

BABY PROVERBS FOR NEW DADS:

One hour's sleep before midnight is all a parent's likely to get.

BABY PROVERBS FOR NEW DADS:

Two's company, then
you have a baby.

BABY PROVERBS FOR NEW DADS:

You can take a baby to the sippy cup, but you cannot make it drink.

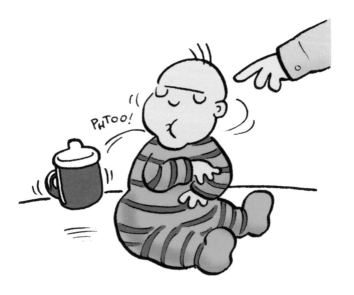

It's an ill wind that needs
the most burping.

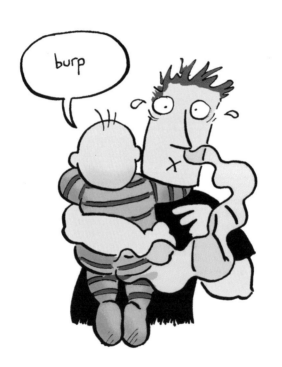

BABY PROVERBS FOR NEW DADS:

Where there's a will,
there's frequently a rather
interesting choice of
baby's name.

THE NEW DAD'S DICTIONARY

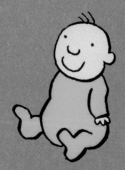

ALLERGY: A few marks that appear on your child that in your day would have just been called spots.

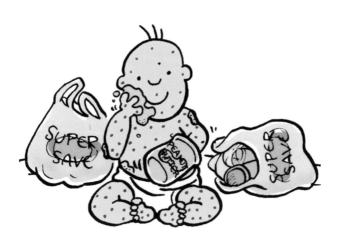

THE NEW DAD'S DICTIONARY:

BURPING: An activity passionately encouraged in children until they are weaned, and thereafter equally passionately discouraged.

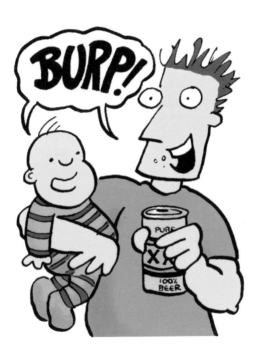

THE NEW DAD'S DICTIONARY:

COITUS INTERRUPTUS:
The effect of children's
Sunday morning television
programmes finishing earlier
than the parents thought.

THE NEW DAD'S DICTIONARY:

CONSTIPATION: A no-go situation. cf. DIARRHOEA: An ongoing situation.

THE NEW DAD'S DICTIONARY:

CONTRACTION: One of the first signs of a baby's arrival. The most notable are contraction of space, social life and spare cash.

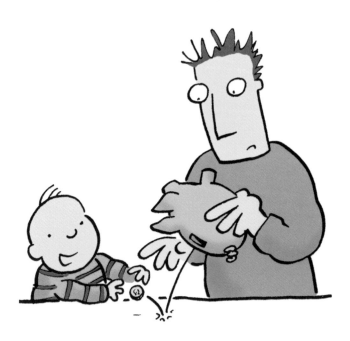

THE NEW DAD'S DICTIONARY:

FAMILY PLANNING:
Keeping rival
grandparents apart.

THE NEW DAD'S DICTIONARY:

HEREDITY: The uncanny reappearance in children of all the good characteristics of one's own family and all the bad characteristics of one's in-laws.

THE NEW DAD'S DICTIONARY:

IRON: A great help to the well-being of the pregnant and nursing mother. cf. IRONING: No help at all to the well-being of the pregnant and nursing mother.

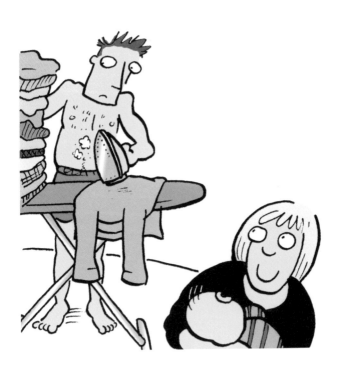

SUPPLEMENTARY FEEDING: Baby's habit of coming into parents' bed on Sunday mornings and eating the newspapers.

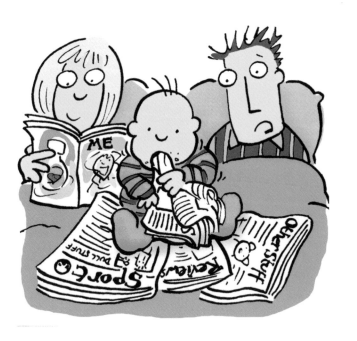

AND REMEMBER...

A baby is yours until it leaves home, but your bank balance will never truly be yours again.

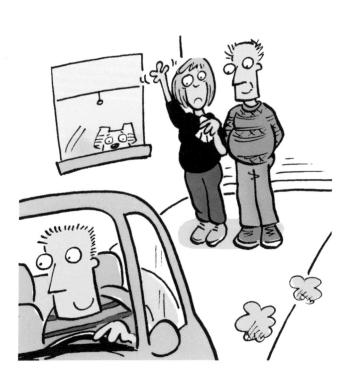

If you're interested in finding out more about our books, find us on Facebook at Summersdale Publishers and follow us on Twitter at @Summersdale.

www.summersdale.com